The Complete Lean and Green Recipe Book

An Amazing Collection of Recipes to Improve Your Meals and Boost Your Appetite

Linda Carey

Table of contents

Strawberry Cheesecake

Prep Time: 15 minutes.

Cook Time: 0 minutes.

Serves: 6

Ingredients:

- 1/2 cup cream cheese
- 2 tablespoons coconut palm sugar
- 1/2 cup Greek yogurt
- 2 teaspoons lemon juice, squeezed
- 1/4 cup strawberry preserves
- 1 cup strawberries diced
- 1/3 cup almonds whole
- 4 dates

Preparation:

1. Beat cream cheese with lemon juice, yogurt, and sugar in a blender for 3 minutes.
2. Mix strawberries with preserves in a small bowl.
3. Grind the almonds with dates in a food processor.

4.   Divide the almond mixture in a muffin tray and press it.
5.   Add cheesecake batter on top and divide the strawberry mixture on top.
6.   Refirgerate these mini cheese cakes for 1 hour.
7.   Serve.

Serving Suggestion: Serve the cheese cakes with creamy frosting on top.

Variation Tip: Add chopped pecans or walnuts to the batter.

Nutritional Information Per Serving:

Calories 195 | Fat 3g |Sodium 355mg | Carbs 20g | Fiber 1g | Sugar 25g | Protein 1g

Coffee Cake Muffins

Prep Time: 15 minutes.

Cook Time: 15 minutes.

Serves: 4

Ingredients:

- 1 packet medifast cappuccino
- 1 packet medifast chocolate chip pancakes
- 1 packet of stevia
- 1 tablespoon egg, beaten
- 1/4 teaspoon baking powder
- 1/4 cup water

Preparation:

1. Mix cappuccino fueling and rest of the ingredients in a bowl until smooth.
2. Divide the mixture into the muffin tray.
3. Bake the muffins for 15 minutes in the oven at 350 degrees F.
4. Allow the muffins to cool and serve.

Serving Suggestion: Serve the muffins with chopped nuts on top.

Variation Tip: Add dried raisins to the muffins.

Nutritional Information Per Serving:

Calories 203 | Fat 8.9g |Sodium 340mg | Carbs 24.7g | Fiber 1.2g | Sugar 11.3g | Protein 5.3g

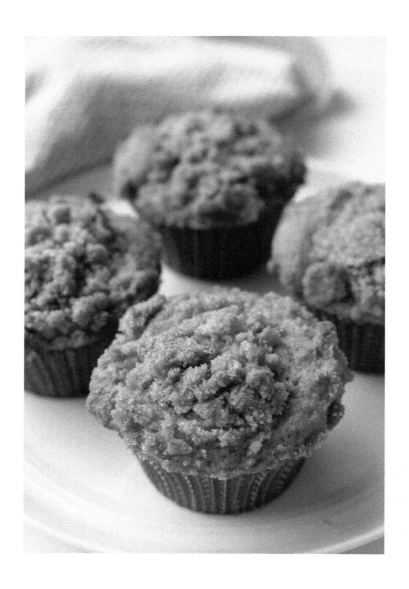

Peanut Butter Balls

Prep Time: 15 minutes.

Cook Time: 0 minutes.

Serves: 4

Ingredients:

- 1 Medifast chocolate pudding
- 1 Medifast chocolate shake
- 4 tablespoons powdered peanut butter
- 2 tablespoons water
- 1/4 cup unsweetened almond milk

Preparation:

1. Mix chocolate pudding and all the ingredients in a bowl.
2. Make 8 fudge balls out of this mixture.
3. Place the fudge balls in a baking sheet and refrigerate for 4 hours.
4. Serve.

Serving Suggestion: Serve the balls with chopped nuts on top.

Variation Tip: Add vanilla extracts to the dessert.

Nutritional Information Per Serving:

Calories 153 | Fat 1g |Sodium 8mg | Carbs 66g | Fiber 0.8g | Sugar 56g | Protein 1g

Brownie in a Tray

Prep Time: 15 minutes.

Cook Time: 1 minutes.

Serves: 4

Ingredients:

- 1 Medifast Brownie Mix
- 3 tablespoons water
- 1 wedge cream cheese
- 2 tablespoons Peanut butter powder
- 1 tablespoon water

Preparation:

6. Blend brownie mix with 3 tbs water in a shallow bowl.

7. Heat this mixture in the microwave for 1 minutes.

8. Slice the cream cheese slices and place on top of the brownie.

9. Blend peanut butter powder with 1 tablespoon water in a bowl.

10. Pour this mixture over the brownie.

11. Serve.

Serving Suggestion: Serve the brownie with chocolate syrup or berries on top.

Variation Tip: Add crushed walnuts or pecans to the brownie.

Nutritional Information Per Serving:

Calories 198 | Fat 14g |Sodium 272mg | Carbs 34g | Fiber 1g | Sugar 9.3g | Protein 1.3g

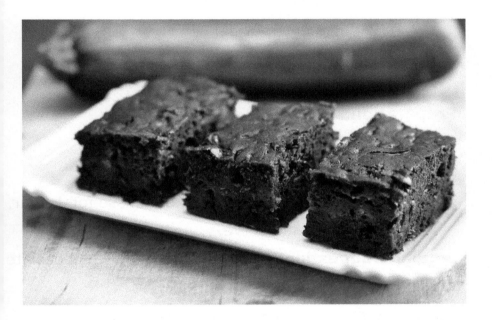

Dark Chocolate Mousse

Prep Time: 10 minutes.

Cook Time: 0 minutes.

Serves: 2

Ingredients:

- 2 ripe avocados, peeled and pitted
- ½ cup dark cocoa powder
- 1 tablespoon vanilla extract
- ¼ cup stevia powder
- ¼ cup almond milk
- 1 pinch salt

Preparation:

1. Blend all avocados with rest of the ingredients in a blender until smooth.
2. Cover and refrigerate the mousse for 1 hour.
3. Garnish and serve.

Serving Suggestion: Serve the mousse with chocolate sauce on top.

Variation Tip: Add crushed nuts or coconut flakes.

Nutritional Information Per Serving:

Calories 159 | Fat 3g |Sodium 277mg | Carbs 21g | Fiber 1g | Sugar 9g | Protein 2g

Banana Pudding

Prep Time: 10 minutes.

Cook Time: 15 minutes.

Serves: 4

Ingredients:

Cookie layer:

- 2 tablespoons butter softened
- 1 teaspoon vanilla extract
- 1 egg
- 1/2 cup almond flour
- 1 teaspoon baking powder
- 1/4 cup erythritol

Pudding layer:

- 2 cups heavy whipping cream
- 1 cup almond milk
- 2 teaspoons vanilla extract
- 6 egg yolks
- 1/2 cup erythritol
- 1 medium banana, sliced

Whipped cream layer:

- 1/2 cup heavy whipping cream
- 1 teaspoon vanilla extract
- 1/4 cup erythritol
- 1/4 teaspoon xanthan gum

Preparation:

1. At 350 degrees F, preheat your oven.
2. Layer a baking sheet with parchment paper.
3. Mix butter with egg and vanilla in a bowl.
4. Stir in baking powder, almond flour and erythritol then mix well.
5. Spread this mixture in an 8x16 inches baking sheet.
6. Bake this batter for 15 minutes until golden brown.
7. Meanwhile, mix all the pudding ingredients in a saucepan and cook until the pudding thickens.
8. Spread the pudding over the baked cookie layer.
9. Beat all the cream layer ingredients in a bowl until fluffy.
10. Spread this mixture over the pudding layer.
11. Cover and refrigerate for 1 hour.
12. Slice and serve.

Serving Suggestion: Serve the pudding cups with peanut butter frosting on top.

Variation Tip: Add chocolate chips or a teaspoon of crushed nuts to the batter for the change of flavor.

Nutritional Information Per Serving:

Calories 268 | Fat 14g |Sodium 122mg | Carbs 23.3g | Fiber 1.2g | Sugar 12g | Protein 6g

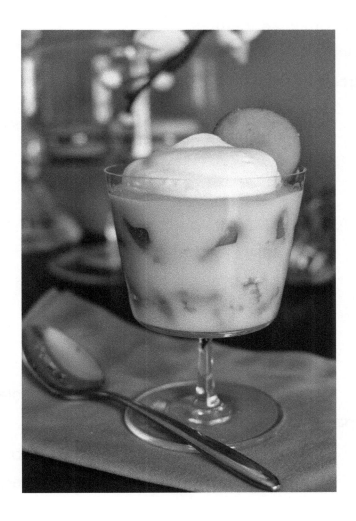

Garlic Chicken with Zoodles

Prep Time: 15 minutes.

Cook Time: 28 minutes.

Serves: 4

Ingredients:

- 1 ½ lbs boneless chicken breasts
- 1 tablespoon olive oil
- 1 cup Greek yogurt
- ½ cup chicken broth
- ½ teaspoons garlic powder
- ½ teaspoons Italian seasoning
- ¼ cup parmesan cheese
- 1 cup spinach, chopped
- 6 sun-dried tomatoes slices
- 1 tablespoon garlic, chopped
- 1 ½ cups zucchini, cut into thin noodles

Preparation:

1. Pat dry the chicken breasts and rub them with cooking oil, black pepper and salt.
2. Sear the chicken in a skillet for 5 minutes per side until golden brown.

3. Transfer this prepared chicken to a plate and keep it aside.
4. Mix parmesan cheese, Italian seasoning, garlic powder, chicken broth and yogurt in a large skillet.
5. Mix and cook this mixture until it thickens.
6. Stir in sun-dried tomatoes and spinach, then cook for 3 minutes.
7. Toss in zucchini noodles and place the chicken on top.
8. At 350 degrees F, preheat your oven.
9. Bake the chicken and zucchini noodles for 15 minutes.
10. Serve warm.

Serving Suggestion: Serve the zoodles with a kale salad on the side.

Variation Tip: Coat the chicken with coconut shreds.

Nutritional Information Per Serving:

Calories 414 | Fat 15g |Sodium 587mg | Carbs 8g | Fiber 1g | Sugar 5g | Protein 60g

Chicken Zucchini Boats

Prep Time: 15 minutes.

Cook Time: 50 minutes.

Serves: 4

Ingredients:

- 4 zucchinis
- 1 lb. ground chicken
- 1/4 teaspoon salt
- 1/4 teaspoon black pepper
- 2 garlic cloves, minced
- 1 cup pasta sauce
- 1/4 cup parmesan cheese, grated
- 1/2 cup mozzarella cheese, shredded
- Sliced fresh basil for topping

Preparation:

1. At 400 degrees F, preheat your oven.
2. Layer a 9x13 inch baking pan with cooking spray.
3. Sauté chicken with black pepper and salt in a skillet for 10 minutes.
4. Add garlic and cook for 1 minute.
5. Stir in pasta sauce and sauté for 3 minutes.
6. Slice each zucchini boat in half, lengthwise and scoop out some flesh from the centre.

7. Divide the chicken into each zucchini half.

8. Place the prepared zucchini boats in the baking dish with cut-side up.

9. Sprinkle parmesan and mozzarella cheese on top.

10. Cover this baking dish with foil and bake for 35 minutes.

11. Sprinkle basil and serve.

Serving Suggestion: Serve the zucchini boats with fresh herbs on top and a bowl of steamed rice.

Variation Tip: Add some chopped bell pepper to the filling.

Nutritional Information Per Serving:

Calories 332 | Fat 18g |Sodium 611mg | Carbs 13.3g | Fiber 0g | Sugar g4 | Protein 38g

Medifast Chicken Fry

Prep Time: 15 minutes.

Cook Time: 10 minutes.

Serves: 4

Ingredients:

- 12 ounces boneless chicken breast
- 1 cup red bell pepper, chopped
- 1 cup green bell pepper, chopped
- 8 ounces broccoli slaw
- 1/2 cup chicken broth
- 2 tablespoons soy sauce
- 1 teaspoon crushed red pepper

Preparation:

1. Sauté broccoli slaw and peppers in a pan with chicken broth.
2. Stir in chicken, red pepper and soy sauce.
3. Cook for 10 minutes with occasional stirring.
4. Serve warm.

Serving Suggestion: Serve the stir fry with roasted green beans.

Variation Tip : Add some sliced onion and spring onion to the fry.

Nutritional Information Per Serving:

Calories 235 | Fat 5g |Sodium 422mg | Carbs 16g |
Fiber 0g | Sugar 1g | Protein 25g

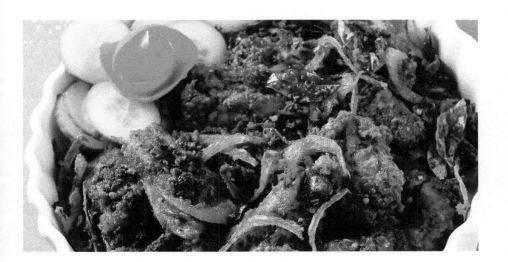

Tuscan Chicken

Prep Time: 15 minutes.

Cook Time: 23 minutes.

Serves: 4

Ingredients:

- 1 lb. boneless chicken breasts, sliced
- 2 tablespoons butter spread
- 4 cups kale leaves, chopped
- 2 garlic cloves, chopped
- 1 package Knorr rice sides cheddar broccoli
- ¼ cup sun-dried tomatoes, sliced
- Lemon wedges

Preparation:

1. Rub the chicken with black pepper and salt.
2. Sear the chicken with 1 tablespoon butter in a skillet for 5 minutes per side.
3. Transfer this prepared chicken to a plate and keep it aside.
4. Sauté garlic and kale with remaining butter in the same skillet over medium-high heat for 3 minutes.
5. Stir in 2 cup water and cheddar broccoli, and tomatoes then cook for 5 minutes with occasional stirring.

6. Return the cooked chicken to the skillet and
    cook for 5 minutes.
7. Garnish with lemon wedges and pine nuts.
8. Enjoy.

Serving Suggestion: Serve the chicken with roasted
veggies.

Variation Tip: Replace kale with baby spinach if
needed.

Nutritional Information Per Serving:

Calories 369 | Fat 14g |Sodium 442mg | Carbs 13.3g |
Fiber 0.4g | Sugar 2g | Protein 32.3g

Chicken Taco Soup

Prep Time: 15 minutes.

Cook Time: 5 hours.

Serves: 4

Ingredients:

- 2 cups chicken broth
- 1/2 teaspoon cumin
- 2 cups of water
- 1 cup Rotel diced tomatoes
- 1 teaspoon taco seasoning
- 1/4 teaspoon chili powder
- 1 garlic clove, minced
- 14 ounces of raw chicken breasts
- 2 cups cabbage, chopped

Preparation:

1. Add all the taco soup ingredients to a crockpot.
2. Cover its lid and cook for 5 hours on low heat.
3. Shred the cooked chicken and return to the soup.
4. Serve warm.

Serving Suggestion: Serve the soup with fresh cucumber and couscous salad.

Variation Tip: Add some canned corn kernels to the soup.

Nutritional Information Per Serving:

 Calories 453 | Fat 2.4g |Sodium 216mg | Carbs 18g | Fiber 2.3g | Sugar 1.2g | Protein 23.2g

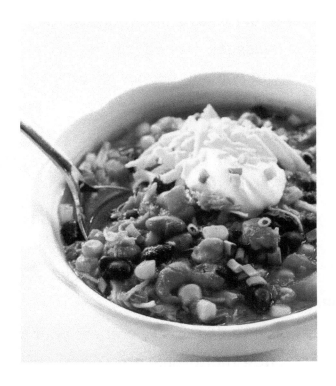

Chicken Chili

Prep Time: 15 minutes.

Cook Time: 35 minutes.

Serves: 8

Ingredients:

- 8 (6 inches) corn tortillas
- 2 teaspoons vegetable oil
- 1 lb boneless chicken breast, diced
- 1 teaspoon ground cumin
- 1 cup poblano pepper, chopped
- 1/2 cup onion, chopped
- 1 garlic clove, minced
- 2 (14 ounces) cans of reduced-fat chicken broth
- 2 (15 ounces) cans of pinto beans
- 1 cups salsa Verde
- 2 tablespoons cilantro, minced

Preparation:

1. At 400 degrees F, preheat your oven.
2. Cut 4 the tortilla into ½ inch strips and toss them with 1 teaspoon oil.
3. Spread the tortillas on a baking sheet and bake for 12 minutes.

4. Grate the remaining tortillas into pieces and keep them aside.
5. Sauté chicken pieces with 1 teaspoon oil and cumin in a skillet for 5 minutes.
6. Transfer this prepared chicken to a plate and keep it aside.
7. Sauté garlic, onion and poblano peppers in the same skillet for 3 minutes.
8. Add grated tortillas, salsa, beans, broth and chicken, then cook for 15 minutes on a simmer.
9. Garnish with cilantro and baked tortillas.
10. Serve warm.

Serving Suggestion: Serve the chili with toasted bread slices.

Variation Tip: Add corn kernels to the chicken chili.

Nutritional Information Per Serving:

Calories 354 | Fat 25g |Sodium 412mg | Carbs 22.3g | Fiber 0.2g | Sugar 1g | Protein 28.3g

Lean Green Chicken Soup

Prep Time: 15 minutes.

Cook Time: 25 minutes.

Serves: 6

Ingredients:

- 2 quarts chicken broth
- 1 1/2 lbs. boneless chicken breast
- 2 celery stalks, chopped
- 2 cups green beans, chopped
- 1 1/2 cups peas
- 2 cups asparagus, chopped
- 1 cup green onions, diced
- 6 garlic cloves, minced
- 2 cups spinach leaves, chopped
- 1 bunch watercress, chopped
- 1/2 cup parsley leaves, chopped
- 1/3 cup basil leaves, chopped
- 1 teaspoon salt
- 1/2 teaspoon black pepper

Preparation:

1. Boil chicken broth in a cooking pot and add chicken breasts.
2. Cook the chicken on a simmer for 15 minutes.

3.   Stir in black pepper, salt, garlic, onions, asparagus, peas, green beans and celery.
4.   Cook this mixture on a simmer for 10 minutes then remove from the heat.
5.   Shred the cooked chicken with a fork.
6.   Add basil, parsley, watercress and spinach to the soup.
7.   Serve warm.

Serving Suggestion: Serve the soup with white rice or sweet potato salad.

Variation Tip: Add some zucchini noodles to the soup.

Nutritional Information Per Serving:

Calories 105 | Fat 15g |Sodium 852mg | Carbs 7g | Fiber 2g | Sugar 2g | Protein 15g

Avocado Chicken Salad

Prep Time: 15 minutes.

Cook Time: 0 minutes.

Serves: 4

Ingredients:

- 10 ounces cooked chicken breasts, sliced
- 1/2 cup Greek yogurt
- 3 ounces avocado, chopped
- 1/2 teaspoon garlic powder
- 1/4 teaspoon salt
- 1/8 teaspoons black pepper
- 1 tablespoon 1 teaspoon lime juice
- 1/4 cup fresh cilantro, chopped

Preparation:

1. Toss chicken with yogurt, avocado and the rest of the ingredients in a salad bowl.
2. Cover and refrigerate for 30 minutes.
3. Serve.

Serving Suggestion: Serve the salad with avocado guacamole on top.

Variation Tip: Add boiled peas to the salad.

Nutritional Information Per Serving:

Calories 352 | Fat 14g |Sodium 220mg | Carbs 16g | Fiber 0.2g | Sugar 1g | Protein 26g

Chicken Pesto Pasta

Prep Time: 15 minutes.

Cook Time: 0 minutes.

Serves: 6

Ingredients:

Kale Pesto

- 3 cups raw kale
- 2 cup fresh basil
- 2 tablespoons olive oil
- 3 tablespoons lemon juice
- 3 garlic cloves
- ¼ teaspoon salt

Pasta Salad

- 2 cups cooked chicken breast, diced
- 6 ounces cooked rotini chickpea pasta
- 1 cup arugula
- 3oz fresh mozzarella, diced

Preparation:

1. Blend kale with all the pesto ingredients in a blender until smooth.
2. Cook chicken cubes with pasta, arugula, pesto and mozzarella in a salad bowl.
3. Serve.

Serving Suggestion: Serve the pasta with a spinach salad.

Variation Tip: Add canned corns to the pasta.

Nutritional Information Per Serving:

 Calories 388 | Fat 8g |Sodium 339mg | Carbs 8g | Fiber 1g | Sugar 2g | Protein 13g

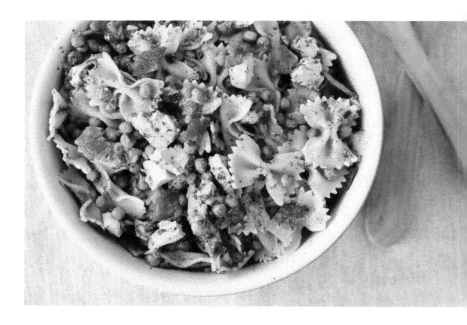

Sesame Chicken Fry

Prep Time: 15 minutes.

Cook Time: 16 minutes.

Serves: 4

Ingredients:

For the sauce:

- 1/3 cup soy sauce
- ⅓ cup of water
- 3 garlic cloves, minced
- 2 tablespoons coconut sugar
- 1 tablespoon sesame oil
- 1 tablespoon rice vinegar
- 1 tablespoon fresh ginger, grated
- 1 tablespoon sesame seeds
- ½ teaspoon red pepper flakes
- ½ tablespoon arrowroot starch

For the chicken:

- 1/2 tablespoon sesame oil
- 1 lb. lean ground chicken
- ½ teaspoon garlic powder
- Salt and black pepper, to taste

For the veggies:

- ½ tablespoon toasted sesame oil
- 2 large carrots, sliced

- 1 white onion, chopped
- 1 red bell pepper, chopped
- 12 ounces green beans, trimmed

For serving

- ½ cup roasted cashews, chopped
- Scallions
- Extra sesame seeds

Preparation:

1. Mix soy sauce, arrowroot starch, red pepper flakes, sesame seeds, ginger, rice vinegar, sesame oil, coconut sugar, garlic, and water in a bowl.
2. Sauté ground chicken with ½ tablespoons sesame oil in a large pot until golden brown.
3. Stir in black pepper, salt and garlic powder.
4. Transfer this meat to a bowl and keep it aside.
5. Sauté onion with carrots and ½ tablespoons sesame oil in the same pan for 4 minutes.
6. Stir in green beans and bell pepper then cook for 8 minutes.
7. Return the chicken to the veggies and cook for 4 minutes.
8. Serve with brown rice or quinoa.

9. Garnish with roasted cashews, scallions and sesame seeds.

10. Enjoy.

Serving Suggestion: Serve the chicken fry with steaming white rice.

Variation Tip: Add roasted peanuts on top.

Nutritional Information Per Serving:

Calories 301 | Fat 16g |Sodium 189mg | Carbs 32g | Fiber 0.3g | Sugar 0.1g | Protein 28.2g

Teriyaki Chicken Broccoli

Prep Time: 15 minutes.

Cook Time: 13 minutes.

Serves: 4

Ingredients:

- 10 ounces chicken strips
- 2 tablespoons teriyaki sauce
- 1 tablespoon fresh garlic, minced
- 1/2 cup yellow onion, diced
- 2 cups broccoli, florets
- 1/4 cup fresh scallions. sliced
- 2 tablespoons water

Preparation:

1. Sauté onion and garlic in a non-stick skillet for 5 minutes.
2. Stir in chicken and the rest of the ingredients, then cook for 8 minutes.
3. Serve warm.

Serving Suggestion: Serve the chicken broccoli with cauliflower rice.

Variation Tip: Add dried herbs to the mixture for seasoning.

Nutritional Information Per Serving:

Calories 231 | Fat 20g |Sodium 941mg | Carbs 30g | Fiber 0.9g | Sugar 1.4g | Protein 14.6g

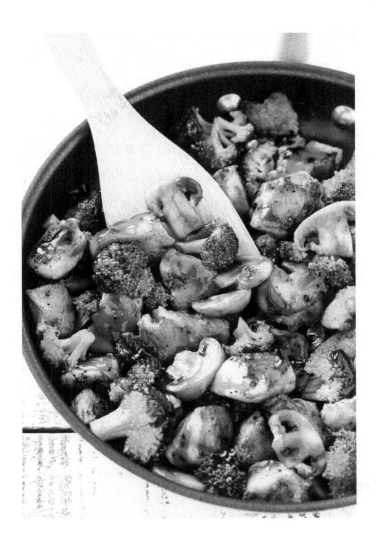

White Chicken Chili

Prep Time: 15 minutes.

Cook Time: 8 hours.

Serves: 6

Ingredients:

- 3 boneless chicken breasts
- 2 (15 ½ ounce) cans great northern beans
- 1 (15 ounce) of sweet golden corn
- 1 (4 ½ ounce) can green chiles, chopped
- 2 (14.5 ounce) cans chicken broth
- 1 sweet yellow onion, chopped
- 3 garlic cloves, minced
- 1 lime, juiced
- 1 teaspoon cumin
- 1/2 teaspoon onion powder
- 1/2 teaspoon garlic powder
- 1 1/2 teaspoon chilli powder
- 1/4 teaspoon cayenne pepper
- Black pepper, to taste
- Paprika, to taste

Preparation:

1. Add chicken, beans and all other ingredients to a crockpot.

2. Cover and cook the chicken chilli for 8 hours on Low.

3. Shred this cooked chicken with two forks and return to the chili.

4. Garnish with your favorite toppings.

5. Enjoy.

Serving Suggestion: Serve the chicken chilli with a fresh crouton's salad.

Variation Tip: Add a drizzle of cheese on top.

Nutritional Information Per Serving:

Calories 300 | Fat 2g |Sodium 374mg | Carbs 30g | Fiber 6g | Sugar 3g | Protein 32g

Chicken Thighs with Green Olive

Prep Time: 15 minutes.

Cook Time: 20 minutes.

Serves: 4

Ingredients:

- 1 ½ lb. boneless chicken thighs, trimmed
- ¼ teaspoon salt
- ¼ teaspoon black pepper
- ¼ cup all-purpose flour
- 3/4 cup cranberry juice
- 1 tablespoon 1 teaspoon olive oil
- 4 garlic cloves, minced
- ¾ cup chicken broth
- 1/4 cup dried cherries
- ¼ cup sliced green olives. pitted
- 2 tablespoons red-wine vinegar
- 1 tablespoon brown sugar
- 1 teaspoon dried oregano

Preparation:

1. Rub the chicken with black pepper and salt, then coat with the flour.
2. Mix ¼ cup cranberry juice with 4 teaspoons flour in a bowl until smooth.

3. Sear the seasoned chicken in 1 tablespoon oil in a skillet over medium heat for 5 minutes per side.

4. Transfer the prepared chicken to a plate and keep them aside.

5. Stir in garlic, 1 teaspoon oil, and sauté for 30 seconds.

6. Add flour juice mixture, ½ cup cranberry juice, cherries, oregano, brown sugar, vinegar and olives.

7. Boil this mixture, reduce the heat, simmer and cook for 6 minutes with occasional stirring.

8. Return this chicken to the pan and cook for 2 minutes.

9. Serve warm.

Serving Suggestion: Serve the chicken with toasted bread slices.

Variation Tip: Add butter sauce on top of the chicken before cooking.

Nutritional Information Per Serving:

Calories 419 | Fat 13g |Sodium 432mg | Carbs 9.1g | Fiber 3g | Sugar 1g | Protein 33g

Chicken Divan

Prep Time: 15 minutes.

Cook Time: 41 minutes.

Serves: 8

Ingredients:

- 2 tablespoons olive oil
- 1 lb. boneless chicken breast, diced
- 1 large onion, diced
- 3 garlic cloves, minced
- ¾ teaspoon salt
- ½ teaspoon black pepper
- ½ teaspoon dry thyme
- ¼ cup dry sherry
- 2 cups chicken broth
- ¼ cup all-purpose flour
- 2/3 cup Parmesan cheese, grated
- ¼ cup sour cream
- 2 pieces Broccoli crowns, chopped
- ½ cup water
- 3 tablespoons panko
- ½ teaspoon paprika

Preparation:

1. At 400 degrees F, preheat your oven.

2. Grease a 2 ½ quart baking dish with cooking spray.

3. Sauté chicken with 1 tablespoon oil in a skillet until golden brown for 10 minutes.

4. Transfer to a plate, cover with a foil and keep aside.

5. Sauté onion, thyme, black pepper, salt and garlic with 2 teaspoons oil in the same skillet for 4 minutes.

6. Stir in sherry then cook a simmer for 3 minutes.

7. Pour in 1 ½ cup broth then cook on a simmer with occasional stirring.

8. Mix flour with ½ cup broth in a bowl and pour into the skillet.

9. Cook until the mixture thickens then add sour cream and 1/3 cup parmesan.

10. Return the chicken to the mixture and mix well

11. Add broccoli and ½ cup water to a bowl, cover and microwave for 2 minutes.

12. Drain and transfer the broccoli to the chicken then mix well.

13. Spread this chicken mixture in the prepared casserole dish.
14. Drizzle remaining parmesan, panko, paprika and 1 teaspoon oil on top.
15. Bake for 22 minutes in the preheated oven.
16. Serve warm.

Serving Suggestion: Serve the chicken divan with roasted veggies on the side.

Variation Tip: Add peas and corn to the casserole.

Nutritional Information Per Serving:

Calories 334 | Fat 16g |Sodium 462mg | Carbs 31g | Fiber 0.4g | Sugar 3g | Protein 35.3g

Spicy Taco Meat

Prep Time: 15 minutes.

Cook Time: 16 minutes.

Serves: 6

Ingredients:

- 8 ounces lean ground beef
- 8 ounces lean ground turkey breast
- ½ cup onion, chopped
- 1 (10-ounce) can dice tomatoes
- ½ teaspoon ground cumin
- 1/2 teaspoon ground chipotle chile
- ½ teaspoon dried oregano

Preparation:

1. Sauté onion, turkey and beef in a skillet over medium heat for 10 minutes.
2. Transfer the mixture to a plate and keep it aside.
3. Stir in tomatoes, oregano, cumin and chipotle.
4. Sauté for 6 minutes then return the meat mixture.
5. Serve warm.

Serving Suggestion: Serve the taco meat with mashed sweet potato and roasted asparagus on the side.

Variation Tip: Use chicken mince instead of beef.

Nutritional Information Per Serving:

Calories 305 | Fat 25g |Sodium 532mg | Carbs 2.3g | Fiber 0.4g | Sugar 2g | Protein 18.3g

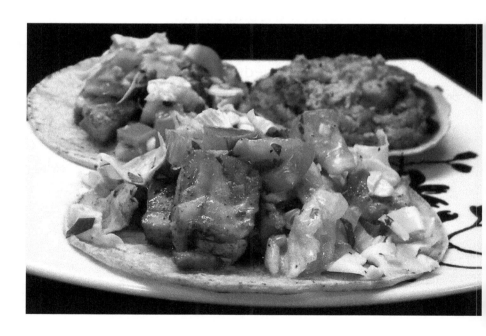

Taco Salad

Prep Time: 15 minutes.

Cook Time: 10 minutes.

Serves: 6

Ingredients:

- 1 lb. lean ground beef
- 1 tablespoon chili powder
- 8 green onions, chopped,
- 1 head romaine lettuce, chopped
- 1 medium tomato, chopped
- 1 avocado, diced
- 1 4-ounce can olives, sliced
- 1 1/2 cups cheddar cheese, grated
- 1/2 cup plain yogurt
- 1/2 cup salsa

Preparation:

1. Sauté beef with black pepper, salt, onions, and chili powder in a skillet until brown.
2. Transfer to a salad bowl then toss in remaining ingredients.
3. Serve.

Serving Suggestion: Serve the salad with toasted bread slices.

Variation Tip: Add crumbled feta cheese on top.

Nutritional Information Per Serving:

Calories 325 | Fat 16g |Sodium 431mg | Carbs 22g | Fiber 1.2g | Sugar 4g | Protein 23g

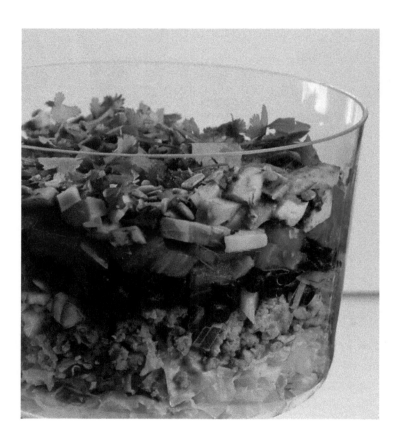

Beef Broccoli

Prep Time: 15 minutes.

Cook Time: 44 minutes.

Serves: 2

Ingredients:

- 1 cup brown rice
- 1 1/2 cups water
- 1/4 cup soy sauce
- 2 tablespoons brown sugar
- 1 tablespoon fresh ginger, grated
- 2 teaspoons rice wine vinegar
- 1 teaspoon sesame oil
- 1 teaspoon sriracha sauce
- 1 tablespoon canola oil
- 1 lb. boneless beef, diced
- 3 garlic cloves, minced
- 2 cups broccoli florets
- 1/4 cup green onions, sliced
- Sesame seeds to garnish

Preparation:

1. Boil rice with water in a pan then cook on low heat for 30 minutes.

2. Mix sriracha, sesame oil. Rice wine vinegar, ginger, brown sugar, and soy sauce in a small bowl.
3. Sauté beef with garlic and oil in a skillet for 10 minutes.
4. Transfer to a plate and keep it aside.
5. Add soy sauce mixture, cooked rice, green onions and broccoli to the same skillet.
6. Cook for 4 minutes then divide in the serving plates.
7. Add meat mixture on top and garnish with sesame seeds.
8. Serve warm.

Serving Suggestion: Serve this beef broccoli with cauliflower rice.

Variation Tip: Add toasted croutons on top.

Nutritional Information Per Serving:

Calories 425 | Fat 14g |Sodium 411mg | Carbs 44g | Fiber 0.3g | Sugar 1g | Protein 28.3g

Beef Bake

Prep Time: 15 minutes.

Cook Time: 35 minutes.

Serves: 6

Ingredients:

- 12 ounces cauliflower rice
- 1 ½ lb lean ground beef
- 15 ounces can of tomato sauce
- ½ cup sour cream
- 1 ¼ cup cottage cheese, shredded
- 2 cups cheddar cheese, shredded
- 1/2 cup green onions, sliced
- 1 teaspoon salt
- 1 teaspoon black pepper

Preparation:

1. At 350 degrees F, preheat your oven.
2. Spread cauliflower rice in a 2 ½ quart baking dish then heat for 5 minutes in the microwave.
3. Sauté beef with oil in a skillet for 10 minutes until brown.
4. Stir in tomato sauce, black pepper and salt.
5. Mix cottage cheese, sour cream, and green onions in a bowl.

6. Spread half of the beef mixture on top cauliflower rice.

7. Top it with half of the cheese mixture then add another layer of beef.

8. Finally add the remaining cheese mixture on top.

9. Bake this casserole for 20 minutes at 350 degrees F, in the preheated oven.

10. Serve warm.

Serving Suggestion: Serve the beef bake with sweet potato salad.

Variation Tip: Add breadcrumbs to the topping for more crispiness.

Nutritional Information Per Serving:

Calories 425 | Fat 15g |Sodium 345mg | Carbs 12.3g | Fiber 1.4g | Sugar 3g | Protein 23.3g

Ground Beef Salad

Prep Time: 15 minutes.

Cook Time: 39 minutes.

Serves: 4

Ingredients:

Taco Ground Beef

- 1 tablespoon olive oil
- 1 ½ lbs lean ground beef
- 1 cup white onion, diced
- ½ cup red bell pepper
- 3 garlic cloves, minced
- 1 teaspoon paprika
- 1 tablespoon onion powder
- 1 teaspoon coriander powder
- 1 teaspoon chili powder
- 1 teaspoon cumin powder
- 1 tablespoon dried oregano
- 1/2 teaspoon cayenne pepper
- Salt and black pepper to taste
- 1 cup chicken broth

Salsa

- 2 medium tomatoes, diced
- ¼ cup red onion, diced
- 1 green bell pepper, diced

- 1 teaspoon jalapeno, chopped
- Fresh cilantro, chopped
- 1 tablespoon lime juice
- 1 small garlic clove, minced
- Salt and pepper to taste

Salad

- 6 cups romaine lettuce, chopped
- ½ avocado, sliced
- lime wedges, for garnish
- Salt and black pepper to taste
- Cilantro for garnish

Preparation:

1. Sauté beef with olive oil in a large pot until brown.
2. Stir in bell pepper and onion then sauté for 8 minutes.
3. Toss in garlic then cook for almost 30 seconds then add all the spices.
4. Mix well then stir in chicken stock ten cook to a boil.
5. Reduce its heat, cover and cook for 30 minutes with occasional stirring.
6. Mix all the salsa ingredients in a bowl, cover and refrigerate for 30 minutes.

7. Toss all lettuces and salad ingredients in a salad bowl.

8. Stir in cooked beef then mix well.

9. Add salsa on top and garnish with cilantro.

10. Enjoy.

Serving Suggestion: Serve the beef salad with roasted asparagus.

Variation Tip: Add a drizzle of parmesan cheese on top.

Nutritional Information Per Serving:

Calories 91 | Fat 5g |Sodium 88mg | Carbs 3g | Fiber 0g | Sugar 0g | Protein 7g

Veggie Beef Stir-Fry

Prep Time: 15 minutes.

Cook Time: 20 minutes.

Serves: 4

Ingredients:

- 12 ounces frozen riced cauliflower
- 1 lb. lean Ground Beef
- 2 tablespoons canola oil
- 1 cup baby Bella mushrooms
- 1 cup green beans, trimmed
- 1 cup matchstick carrots
- 2 garlic cloves, minced
- ¼ cup soy sauce
- ¼ cup teriyaki sauce
- 1 tablespoon brown sugar

Preparation:

1. Add cauliflower rice to a bowl and heat in the microwave for 2 minutes then drain.
2. Sauté beef with cooking oil in a skillet for 10 minutes then remove from the heat.
3. Add mushrooms, garlic, carrots, and green beans then sauté for 5 minutes.
4. Stir in brown sugar, teriyaki sauce and soy sauce then cook for 3 minutes.

5.   Serve warm with cauliflower rice.

Serving Suggestion: Serve the stir fry with cauliflower rice.

Variation Tip: Add a layer of the boiled zucchini noodles to the stir fry.

Nutritional Information Per Serving:

 Calories 276 | Fat 21g |Sodium 476mg | Carbs 12g | Fiber 3g | Sugar 4g | Protein 10g

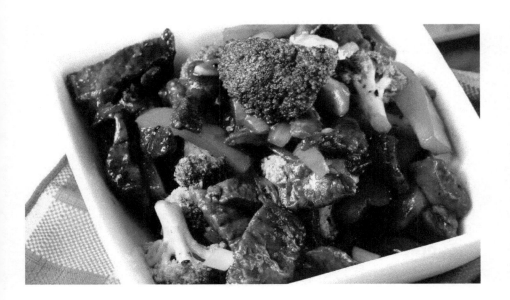

Ground Beef Over Zoodles

Prep Time: 15 minutes.

Cook Time: 11 minutes.

Serves: 4

Ingredients:

Meat

- 1 lb lean ground beef
- 1 small onion, chopped
- 1 garlic clove, chopped
- 1 jalapeno pepper, chopped
- 1/2 teaspoon salt
- 1/2 teaspoon black pepper
- 1/2 teaspoon onion powder
- 1/2 teaspoon smoked paprika
- 1/2 teaspoon ground coriander
- 1 teaspoon dried oregano
- 1/2 cup bone broth
- 1 medium tomato, chopped

Zoodles

- 2 zucchinis, spiralized
- 1/4 teaspoon salt
- 1/4 teaspoon black pepper
- 1/4 teaspoon garlic powder
- 1/2 teaspoon dried oregano

Preparation:

1. Sauté ground beef with black pepper, and salt in a cooking pot for 8 minutes until brown.
2. Stir in jalapeno pepper, garlic and onion then sauté for 1 minute.
3. Add spices and water then cook for 1 minute then add tomato.
4. Transfer the mixture to a plate then add zucchini noodles.
5. Stir in garlic powder, black pepper and salt then sauté for 30 seconds.
6. Serve warm.

Serving Suggestion: Serve the beef zoodles with a fresh green's salad.

Variation Tip: Add chopped herbs on top.

Nutritional Information Per Serving:

Calories 487 | Fat 24g |Sodium 686mg | Carbs 17g | Fiber 1g | Sugar 1.2g | Protein 52g

Mediterranean Beef and Rice

Prep Time: 15 minutes.

Cook Time: 14 minutes.

Serves: 4

Ingredients:

- 10 ounces lean ground beef
- 1/2 cup rice, rinsed and drained
- 1 onion, chopped
- 1 garlic clove, minced
- 1 tablespoon olive oil
- 1 small tomato, chopped
- 1 teaspoon cumin
- 1 teaspoon coriander
- 1 teaspoon mint
- 1 teaspoon paprika
- 1 cup green beans

Preparation:

1. Sauté beef with oil in a skillet for 3 minutes then add paprika, mint, coriander and cumin.
2. Mix well and toss in garlic and onion.
3. Sauté for 1 minute then add 1/3 cup water, a pinch of salt and rice.
4. Cover this pan and cook for 10 minutes on a simmer.

5. Stir in tomato and green beans then cook until the rice is done.

6. Garnish as desired and serve warm.

Serving Suggestion: Serve the beef rice with sweet potato salad.

Variation Tip: Drizzle parmesan cheese on top before serving.

Nutritional Information Per Serving:

Calories 255 | Fat 12g |Sodium 66mg | Carbs 13g | Fiber 2g | Sugar 4g | Protein 22g

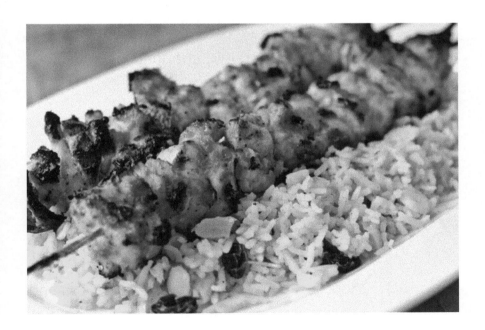

Beef Stew with Green Beans

Prep Time: 15 minutes.

Cook Time: 2 hours.

Serves: 8

Ingredients:

- 6 tablespoons olive oil
- 4 ½ lbs. lean beef stew, cut into cubes
- 3 ½ lbs. green beans
- 1 large onion, minced
- 3 garlic cloves, minced
- 1 large ripe tomato, grated
- 3 tablespoons tomato paste
- 2 tablespoons olive oil
- 1 handful of parsley, chopped
- 2 dried bay leaves
- Salt and black pepper, to taste

Preparation:

1. Sauté meat with olive oil in a cooking pot over high heat until brown.
2. Transfer the meat to a plate and keep it aside.
3. Add garlic and onion to the same pot and sauté until soft.

4. Stir in grated tomato, tomato paste and 1 cup water.

5. Mix this well then return the meat to the pot and cover with enough water.

6. Cook this mixture for 1 hour until meat is tender.

7. Stir in bay leaves, black pepper, salt, parsley and green beans.

8. Cook for 1 hour more hour and serve warm.

Serving Suggestion: Serve the beef stew with fresh herbs on top.

Variation Tip: Add butter to the meat before serving.

Nutritional Information Per Serving:

Calories 405 | Fat 22.7g |Sodium 227mg | Carbs 26.1g | Fiber 1.4g | Sugar 0.9g | Protein 45.2g

Ground Beef Skillet

Prep Time: 15 minutes.

Cook Time: 70 minutes.

Serves: 4

Ingredients:

- 1 spaghetti squash
- 2 teaspoons olive oil
- Salt, black pepper, and garlic powder to taste
- 1 lb. lean ground beef
- 1 small onion, diced
- 1 bell pepper, diced
- 3 garlic cloves, minced
- 1 cup baby Bella mushrooms, chopped
- 2 (15 ounces) canned diced tomatoes
- 1 (15 ounces) can of tomato sauce
- 1 tablespoon Italian seasoning
- Salt and black pepper to taste
- 1/4 cup basil, chopped
- 2 tablespoons parmesan cheese

Preparation:

1. At 400 degrees F, preheat your oven.
2. Cut the prepared squash in half; lengthwise, remove the seed and rub it with garlic powder, black pepper, salt and olive oil.

3. Place the cut squash with the skin side down in a baking sheet and roast for 40 minutes in the preheated oven.
4. Scrap out the roasted squash with a fork and transfer to a plate.
5. Sauté beef in a skillet until brown.
6. Stir in pepper and onion, then sauté for 5 minutes.
7. Add garlic, mushrooms, black pepper and salt, then sauté for 5 minutes.
8. Stir in Italian seasoning, tomato sauce and diced tomatoes.
9. Cook for 20 minutes, then garnish with parsley.
10. Serve the beef on top of the spaghetti squash.
11. Enjoy.

Serving Suggestion: Serve the beef with sautéed carrots on the side.

Variation Tip: Drizzle parmesan cheese on top before serving.

Nutritional Information Per Serving:

Calories 345 | Fat 36g |Sodium 272mg | Carbs 41g | Fiber 0.2g | Sugar 0.1g | Protein 22.5g

Steak with Onions

Prep Time: 15 minutes.

Cook Time: 12 minutes.

Serves: 2

Ingredients:

- 5 ounces lean beef steak
- 1 small onion
- 1 small tomato, halved
- 1 cup spinach
- 1 teaspoon rosemary
- 1 teaspoon olive oil
- Salt and black pepper to taste

Preparation:

1. Sauté onion with oil in a large skillet until soft.
2. Stir in rosemary, and sauté until brown.
3. Add tomato to the skillet and steak to the skillet.
4. Cook for 9 minutes and flip the steaks once cooked halfway through.
5. Add spinach to the steaks and cook for 3 minutes.
6. Serve warm.

Serving Suggestion: Serve the steaks with sautéed green beans and mashed sweet potatoes.

Variation Tip: Drizzle parmesan cheese on top before cooking.

Nutritional Information Per Serving:

Calories 395 | Fat 9.5g |Sodium 655mg | Carbs 13.4g | Fiber 0.4g | Sugar 0.4g | Protein 28.3g

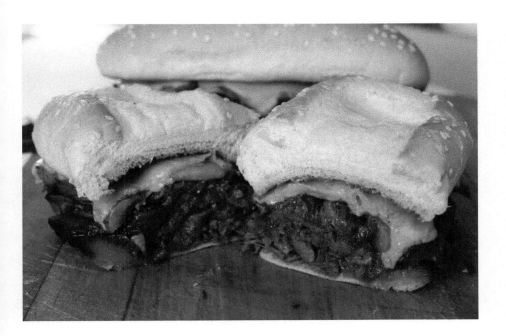

Meatloaf

Prep Time: 15 minutes.

Cook Time: 9 minutes.

Serves: 6

Ingredients:

- 1 onion
- 1 ½ lbs of extra lean ground beef
- 1 cup zucchini, shredded
- ¾ cup green pepper diced
- 1 egg
- 5 teaspoons Worcestershire sauce
- 3 teaspoons grainy mustard
- 2 tablespoons ketchup
- ½ cup breadcrumb
- 1 teaspoon smoked paprika
- ½ teaspoons salt
- ½ teaspoons black pepper

Preparation:

1.   At 375 degrees F, preheat your oven.
2.   Beat egg with black pepper, paprika, salt, Worcestershire sauce, and mustard in a large bowl.
3.   Stir in breadcrumbs and vegetables.

4.   Add beef, mix well and spread this meat mixture into a loaf pan.

5.   Cover the meat mixture with ketchup on top.

6.   Bake the meatloaf for 9 minutes in the oven.

7.   Slice and serve warm.

Serving Suggestion: Serve the meatloaf with fresh green and mashed sweet potatoes.

Variation Tip: Skip zucchini and replace it with an equal amount of shredded carrot.

Nutritional Information Per Serving:

Calories 301 | Fat 5g |Sodium 340mg | Carbs 24.7g | Fiber 1.2g | Sugar 1.3g | Protein 15.3g

BBQ Beef with Sweet Potato Salad

Prep Time: 15 minutes.

Cook Time: 10 hours 8 minutes.

Serves: 4

Ingredients:

For the BBQ Beef:

- 2 lbs. top round beef, diced
- 1 large onion, chopped
- 28 ounces canned tomato puree
- 1 tablespoon chilli powder
- 1 tablespoon dried thyme
- 1/2 teaspoon garlic powder
- 1/2 teaspoon black pepper

Sweet Potato Salad

- 1 1/2 lb. sweet potatoes, diced
- 2 stalk celery, chopped
- 2 green onions, chopped
- 2 tablespoon light mayonnaise
- 1/3 cup fat-free, plain yogurt
- 2 teaspoon apple cider vinegar
- 1/8 teaspoon black pepper

Preparation:

1. Mix all the BBQ beef ingredients in a large bowl.

2. Transfer this mixture to a slow cooker, cover and cook for 10 hours on low heat setting.

3. Meanwhile, cook chopped sweet potatoes with water for 8 minutes until soft.

4. Drain and toss the boiled sweet potatoes with the remaining salad ingredients in a bowl.

5. Serve the BBQ beef with the sweet potatoes.

6. Enjoy.

Serving Suggestion: Serve the beef with roasted green beans.

Variation Tip: Add barbecue sauce to the beef.

Nutritional Information Per Serving:

Calories 448 | Fat 23g |Sodium 350mg | Carbs 18g | Fiber 6.3g | Sugar 1g | Protein 40.3g

Green Beans with Pork and Potatoes

Prep Time: 15 minutes.

Cook Time: 22 minutes.

Serves: 4

Ingredients:

- 1 lb. lean pork, cubed
- 1 large onion, chopped
- 1/2 cup olive oil
- 2 carrots, sliced
- 2 celery sticks, sliced
- 3 fresh tomatoes, grated
- 1 lb. green beans
- 2 potatoes, peeled and cut into quarters
- 1/2 teaspoon salt
- 1/2 teaspoon black pepper

Preparation:

1. Sauté pork with oil in an Pressure Pot for 5 minutes on a Sauté mode.

2. Stir in all the veggies and the rest of the ingredients.

3. Cover the lid and cook on a Manual Setting for 17 minutes.

4. Once done, release the pressure completely, then remove the lid.

5.   Serve warm.

Serving Suggestion: Serve the pork with toasted bread slices.

Variation Tip: Replace potatoes with sweet potatoes.

Nutritional Information Per Serving:

Calories 309 | Fat 25g |Sodium 463mg | Carbs 9.9g | Fiber 0.3g | Sugar 0.3g | Protein 18g

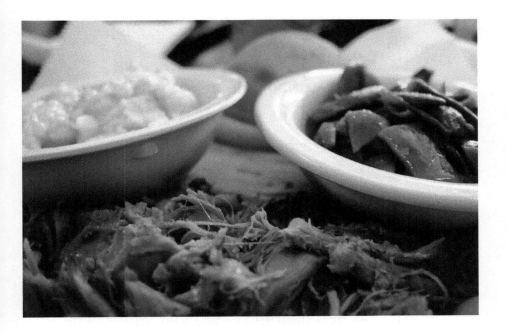

Roasted Pork Chops

Prep Time: 15 minutes.

Cook Time: 16 minutes.

Serves: 6

Ingredients:

- 1 ½ teaspoons paprika
- 1 ½ teaspoons dried ginger
- 1 ½ teaspoons dried mustard
- 1 ½ teaspoons kosher salt
- 1 ½ teaspoons ground black pepper
- 1 ½ tablespoons olive oil
- 6 thick-cut bone-in pork chops

Ginger Green Beans

- 1 ½ tablespoons olive oil
- 2 lb. green beans, de-stemmed
- 1/4 teaspoon crushed red pepper flakes
- 1 teaspoon dried ginger
- 3 teaspoons soy sauce

Preparation:

1. At 500 degrees F, preheat your oven.

2. Mix paprika, black pepper, brown sugar, kosher salt, dried mustard and 1 teaspoon dried ginger in a bowl.

3. Rub the pork chops with the spice rub mixture.

4. Preheat a skillet with 1 tablespoon oil over high heat.

5. Sear the pork chops for almost 2 minutes per side.

6. Roast these chops 6 minutes in the oven, and flip once cooked halfway through.

7. Meanwhile, sauté green beans with 1 tablespoon olive oil in a skillet for 1 minute.

8. Stir in red pepper flakes, soy sauce, ½ teaspoons dried ginger and cook for 5 minutes.

9. Serve the cooked pork chops with the green beans.

10. Enjoy.

Serving Suggestion: Serve the pork chops with roasted green beans.

Variation Tip: Add paprika for more spice.

Nutritional Information Per Serving:

Calories 537 | Fat 20g |Sodium 719mg | Carbs 25.1g | Fiber 0.9g | Sugar 1.4g | Protein 37.8g

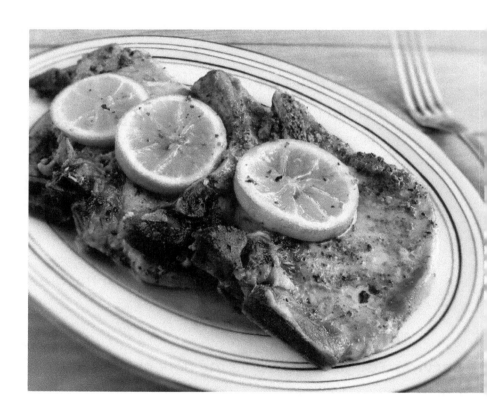

Roasted Shrimp and Green Beans

Prep Time: 15 minutes.

Cook Time: 20 minutes.

Serves: 4

Ingredients:

For the beans:

- 1 lb. green beans, chopped
- 1 tablespoon olive oil
- ½ teaspoons ground coriander
- ½ teaspoons ground cumin
- ¼ teaspoons kosher salt
- ½ teaspoons black pepper
- 1/8 teaspoons Cayenne pepper

For the shrimp:

- 1 lb. raw shrimp, peeled
- 1 tablespoon olive oil
- zest from one lemon
- 1/4 teaspoon salt
- 1/2 teaspoon black pepper

Preparation:

1. At 425 degrees F, preheat your oven.
2. Toss beans with cayenne pepper, black pepper, salt, cumin, coriander, and olive oil in a bowl.

3.   Toss shrimp with black pepper, salt, lemon zest, and oil in another bowl.

4.   Grease a baking sheet with oil and spread the green beans in this sheet.

5.   Roast these beans for 10 minutes, toss and add shrimp on top.

6.   Continue baking for 10 minutes.

7.   Garnish with lemon quarters.

8.   Serve warm.

Serving Suggestion: Serve the shrimp with cauliflower rice risotto.

Variation Tip: Add paprika for more spice.

Nutritional Information Per Serving:

Calories 212 | Fat 9g |Sodium 353mg | Carbs 8g | Fiber 3g | Sugar 4g | Protein 25g

Shrimp Scampi

Prep Time: 15 minutes.

Cook Time: 14 minutes.

Serves: 6

Ingredients:

- 2 tablespoons butter
- 1/2 cup onion, diced
- 3 garlic cloves, minced
- 1 teaspoon dried oregano
- 1 teaspoon dried basil
- 1 teaspoon cayenne pepper
- 1 lb. raw shrimp, peeled and deveined
- 3 tablespoons fresh parsley
- Squeeze of lemon

Preparation:

1. Sauté garlic, spices and onion with butter in a skillet for 7 minutes.
2. Stir in shrimp and sauté for 4 minutes.
3. Add lemon juice and parsley.
4. Serve warm.

Serving Suggestion: Serve the scampi with zucchini noodles.

Variation Tip: Add mixed chopped herbs and lemon zest to the scampi.

Nutritional Information Per Serving:

Calories 376 | Fat 17g |Sodium 1127mg | Carbs 24g | Fiber 1g | Sugar 3g | Protein 29g

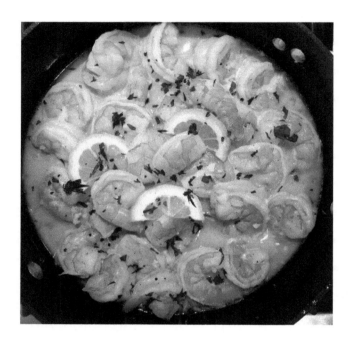

Grilled Shrimp Kabobs

Prep Time: 15 minutes.

Cook Time: 10 minutes.

Serves: 4

Ingredients:

- ¼ cup lemon juice
- ¼ cup vegetable oil
- 1 tablespoon thyme, chopped
- ¼ teaspoon salt
- ¼ teaspoon pepper
- ¾ lb. sea scallops
- 12 large uncooked shrimp
- 8 medium whole fresh mushrooms
- 8 cherry tomatoes
- 1 medium zucchini, cut into slices

Preparation:

1. Set a grill over medium heat.
2. Mix lemon juice with black pepper, salt, oil and thyme in a bowl.
3. Cut all the scallops in half.
4. Thread scallops, zucchini, tomatoes, shrimp and mushrooms on the skewers alternately.
5. Brush the skewers with a lemon juice mixture.

6. Grill these skewers for 10 minutes while basting with lemon mixture and turning the skewers around.

7. Serve warm.

Serving Suggestion: Serve the shrimp skewers with fresh greens on the side.

Variation Tip: Roll the shrimp and scallops in breadcrumbs for a crispy touch.

Nutritional Information Per Serving:

Calories 457 | Fat 19g |Sodium 557mg | Carbs 19g | Fiber 1.8g | Sugar 1.2g | Protein 32.5g

Goan Fish Curry

Prep Time: 15 minutes.

Cook Time: 11 minutes.

Serves: 2

Ingredients:

- 3 garlic cloves, chopped
- 3 cm ginger, chopped
- 1 green chilli, chopped
- 2 tomatoes, chopped
- 1 tablespoon coconut oil
- 1 red onion, diced
- 1 tablespoon garam masala
- 1 tablespoon ground cumin
- 1 x 400ml tin coconut milk
- 1 lb. haddock fillet, cut into chunks
- Juice of 1 lime
- ½ bunch of coriander, chopped

Preparation:

1. Blend tomatoes with chilli, ginger and garlic in a food processor until smooth.
2. Sauté onion with oil in a wok for 2 minutes.
3. Stir in cumin and garam masala then cook for 30 seconds.

4. Add the tomato mixture and coconut milk then boil the mixture.

5. Reduce the heat, and cook for 2 minutes on a simmer.

6. Place the haddock pieces in the curry, cook for 6 minutes on a simmer.

7. Garnish with coriander and lime juice.

8. Serve warm.

Serving Suggestion: Serve the curry with cauliflower rice.

Variation Tip: Replace haddock with codfish if needed.

Nutritional Information Per Serving:

Calories 392 | Fat 16g |Sodium 466mg | Carbs 3.9g | Fiber 0.9g | Sugar 0.6g | Protein 48g

Fish Pie

Prep Time: 15 minutes.

Cook Time: 37 minutes.

Serves: 4

Ingredients:

- 3/4-pint semi-skimmed milk
- 2 bay leaves
- 3 spring onions, chopped
- 3 tablespoons corn flour
- 1 teaspoon Dijon mustard
- 2 tablespoons dill, chopped
- 5 ½ ounces cod, cut into chunks
- 5 ½ ounces smoked haddock, cut into chunks
- 5 ½ ounces salmon, cut into chunks
- 5 ounces raw king prawns
- 3 ½ ounces frozen peas
- 2 potatoes, peeled
- 2 tablespoons olive oil
- 1-ounce vintage Cheddar, grated
- Steamed broccoli, to serve

Preparation:

1. At 350 degrees F, preheat your oven.
2. Boil milk with spring onion and bay leaves in a cooking pot.

3. Mix corn flour with 3 tablespoons cold water in a bowl.

4. Pour into the milk and cook for 4 minutes with occasional stirring until thickens.

5. Stir in dill, and mustard then cook for 2 minutes then discard the bay leaves.

6. Add prawns, peas and fish mix, spread this mixture in a casserole dish.

7. Boil potatoes in salted water for 1 minute then grate them.

8. Mix grated potatoes with olive oil, cheese and seasoning in a bowl.

9. Spread these potatoes on top of the seafood mixture.

10. Bake this pie for 30 minutes in the oven until golden brown.

11. Serve warm.

Serving Suggestion: Serve the fish pie with cauliflower salad.

Variation Tip: Add some cream cheese to the pie filling.

Nutritional Information Per Serving:

Calories 321 | Fat 7.4g |Sodium 356mg | Carbs 9.3g | Fiber 2.4g | Sugar 5g | Protein 37.2g

Parmesan Shrimp Zoodles

Prep Time: 15 minutes.

Cook Time: 18 minutes.

Serves: 4

Ingredients:

- 16 ounces medium shrimp
- 1 cup cherry tomatoes, cut in half
- 8 cups zucchini noodles
- 3 tablespoons olive oil
- 2 tablespoons garlic, minced
- 1/2 cup Parmesan cheese, grated
- 1 teaspoon dried oregano
- 1/2 teaspoon chili powder
- 1/2 teaspoon salt
- 1/2 teaspoon black pepper

Preparation:

1. At 400 degrees F, preheat your oven.
2. Layer a baking sheet with foil sheet.
3. Rinse the shrimp in a colander and leave for 5 minutes.
4. Mix parmesan cheese with black pepper, salt, chili powder, and oregano in a bowl.
5. Drain the shrimp and toss with 1 tablespoon garlic and 1 tablespoon oil in a bowl.

6.   Drizzle half of the cheese mixture on top of the shrimp.

7.   Mix well and drizzle the remaining cheese on top.

8.   Spread the shrimp on the baking sheet and bake for 10 minutes.

9.   Sauté garlic with remaining oil, zucchini noodles and tomatoes in a skillet for 8 minutes.

10.   Serve the shrimp with zucchini noodles and garnish with parmesan cheese.

Serving Suggestion: Serve the shrimp noodles with sautéed vegetables.

Variation Tip: Add canned corn to the shrimp.

Nutritional Information Per Serving:

Calories 258 | Fat 9g |Sodium 994mg | Carbs 1g | Fiber 0.4g | Sugar 3g | Protein 16g

Shrimp and Cauliflower Grits with Greens

Prep Time: 15 minutes.

Cook Time: 20 minutes.

Serves: 4

Ingredients:

Cauliflower Grits

- 1 head cauliflower
- 2 tablespoons avocado oil
- 1 cup of coconut milk
- 1/2 teaspoon sea salt
- 1 tablespoon tapioca starch
- 2 tablespoons water
- 1/2 cup white cheddar, grated

Sautéed Greens

- 1 tablespoon avocado oil
- 4 green onions, sliced
- 4 cups mixed greens
- 1 roasted red pepper, chopped
- Sea salt to taste

Cajun Shrimp:

- 2 strips bacon, sliced
- 2 teaspoons Cajun seasoning
- 1/2 lb. shrimp, peeled and deveined
- Salt to taste

Preparation:

1. Grate the cauliflower in a food processor.
2. Sauté cauliflower with avocado oil in a skillet for 2 minutes.
3. Stir in coconut milk, cover and cook for 10 minutes on low heat.
4. Mix tapioca starch with water and salt in a bowl and add to the cauliflower.
5. Cook the mixture until creamy with occasional stirring.
6. Sauté greens with oil, green onions, red pepper flakes and salt in a skillet for 3 minutes then transfer to a plate.
7. Sauté bacon in a skillet until crispy then add shrimp, Cajun seasoning, green onions and salt.
8. Sauté for 3 minutes then add ¼ cup water.
9. Cook for 2 minutes then serve the shrimp with greens and cauliflower grits.
10. Enjoy.

Serving Suggestion: Serve the shrimp with lemon slices on top.

Variation Tip: Use white pepper for a change of flavor.

Nutritional Information Per Serving:

Calories 378 | Fat 21g |Sodium 146mg | Carbs 7.1g | Fiber 0.1g | Sugar 0.4g | Protein 23g

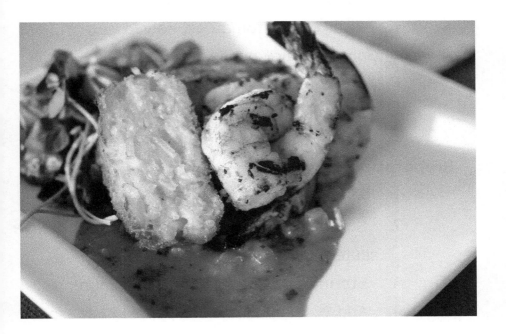

Salmon with Cherry Tomatoes

Prep Time: 15 minutes.

Cook Time: 31 minutes.

Serves: 4

Ingredients:

- 1 cup sweet onion, chopped
- 2 teaspoons garlic, minced
- 2 cups cherry tomatoes, halved
- Salt and black pepper, to taste
- 1 ½ tablespoon balsamic vinegar
- 1 1/2 tablespoon basil leaves, julienned
- 1 (2-lbs.) salmon fillet, cut into 4 pieces

Preparation:

1. At 425 degrees F, preheat your oven.
2. Sauté onion with 3 tablespoons olive oil in a sauté pan for 5 minutes.
3. Stir in garlic then sauté for 1 minute.
4. Add ½ teaspoons black pepper, 1 teaspoon salt and tomatoes then cook for 15 minutes with occasional stirring.
5. Stir in basil and vinegar then mix well.
6. Sear the salmon with olive oil in a skillet for 5 minutes per side.

7. Add the tomato mixture on top of the salmon.

8. Serve warm.

Serving Suggestion: Serve the salmon with fresh greens.

Variation Tip: Drizzle cheddar cheese on top for a rich taste.

Nutritional Information Per Serving:

Calories 351 | Fat 4g |Sodium 236mg | Carbs 19.1g | Fiber 0.3g | Sugar 0.1g | Protein 36g

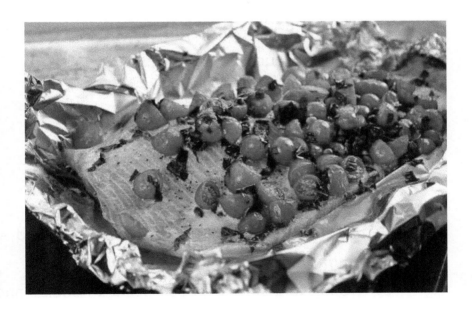

Zucchini Shrimp Scampi

Prep Time: 15 minutes.

Cook Time: 5 minutes.

Serves: 4

Ingredients:

- 2 tablespoons unsalted butter
- 1 lb. shrimp, peeled and deveined
- 3 garlic cloves, minced
- 1/2 teaspoon red pepper flakes
- 1/4 cup chicken stock
- Juice of 1 lemon
- Salt and black pepper, to taste
- 1 1/2 lbs. zucchini, spiralized
- 2 tablespoons Parmesan, grated
- 2 tablespoons parsley leaves, chopped

Preparation:

1. Sauté shrimp with butter, garlic and red pepper flakes in a skillet for 3 minutes.
2. Add chicken stock, black pepper, salt, and lemon juice.
3. Cook to a simmer, add zucchini noodles and cook for 2 minutes.
4. Garnish with parsley and parmesan.
5. Serve warm.

Serving Suggestion: Serve the shrimp zucchini scampi with sweet potato salad.

Variation Tip: Add some chopped bell pepper to the meal.

Nutritional Information Per Serving:

Calories 378 | Fat 7g |Sodium 316mg | Carbs 16.2g | Fiber 0.3g | Sugar 0.3g | Protein 26g

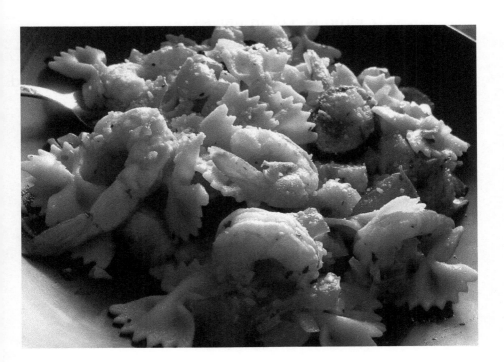

Lemon White Fish Fillets

Prep Time: 15 minutes.

Cook Time: 10 minutes.

Serves: 2

Ingredients:

- 16 ounces cod fillets halibut
- 3 tablespoons olive oil
- 1/4 teaspoon kosher salt
- 1/4 teaspoon black pepper
- 2 lemons, cut in halves

Preparation:

1. Rub the cod fillets with oil, black pepper and oil in a skillet.
2. Cook this codfish for 2 minutes per side.
3. Drizzle lemon juice on top and cook for 3 minutes per side.
4. Enjoy.

Serving Suggestion: Serve the fish with roasted broccoli florets.

Variation Tip: Drizzle lemon zest on top before cooking.

Nutritional Information Per Serving:

Calories 415 | Fat 15g |Sodium 634mg | Carbs 14.3g | Fiber 1.4g | Sugar 1g | Protein 23.3g

Salmon with Herb Garlic Sauce

Prep Time: 15 minutes.

Cook Time: 15 minutes.

Serves: 4

Ingredients:

For the sauce

- 2 garlic cloves, grated
- 3 tablespoons parsley, chopped
- Zest of 1/2 lemon
- Juice of 1/2 lemon
- 3 tablespoons olive oil
- 1/2 teaspoon sea salt

Rest

- 1 tablespoon coconut oil
- 4 salmon fillets
- 12 Brussels sprouts, halved
- 14 asparagus spear, ends cut off
- 1 bunch of broccolini florets
- Olive oil, sea salt, black pepper and lemon

Preparation:

1. At 400 degrees F, preheat your oven.
2. Mix garlic with parsley, lemon juice and zest, and salt in a bowl.

3.   Grease a large roast pan with olive oil and set the salmon in it.

4.   Spread the lemon juice mixture on top of the salmon.

5.   Add the veggies around the salmon and drizzle lemon juice, black pepper and salt on top.

6.   Bake the prepared salmon for 15 minutes in the oven.

7.   Serve warm.

Serving Suggestion: Serve these fish with toasted bread slices.

Variation Tip: Add garlic salt to the seasoning for more taste.

Nutritional Information Per Serving:

Calories 251 | Fat 17g |Sodium 723mg | Carbs 21g | Fiber 2.5g | Sugar 2g | Protein 7.3g

Baked Lemon Garlic Cod

Prep Time: 15 minutes.

Cook Time: 15 minutes.

Serves: 4

Ingredients:

- 4 (6-ounce) boneless cod fillets
- Sea salt, to taste
- Black pepper, to taste
- 1 1/2 teaspoon unsalted butter
- 1 tablespoon olive oil
- 2 garlic cloves, crushed
- 2 tablespoons lemon juice
- 2 tablespoons parsley, chopped

Preparation:

1. At 400 degrees F, preheat your oven.
2. Grease a baking sheet with cooking oil.
3. Rub the cod pieces with black pepper and salt.
4. Sauté garlic with butter in a skillet for 1 minute.
5. Stir in lemon juice and parsley then mix well.
6. Place the cod pieces in the baking sheet and top them with a garlic mixture.
7. Bake the fish for 14 minutes in the oven.

8. Serve warm.

Serving Suggestion: Serve the fish with roasted broccoli florets.

Variation Tip: Add olives or sliced mushrooms around the fish.

Nutritional Information Per Serving:

Calories 246 | Fat 15g |Sodium 220mg | Carbs 40.3g | Fiber 2.4g | Sugar 1.2g | Protein 12.4g

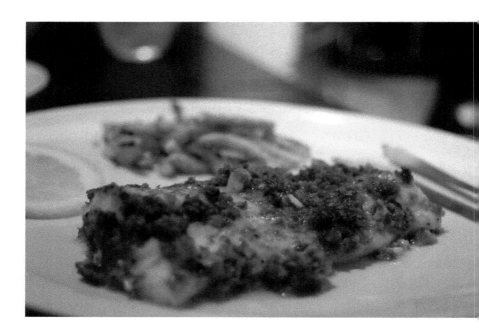

Zucchini Ravioli

Prep Time: 20 minutes.

Cook Time: 30 minutes.

Serves: 6

Ingredients:

- 1 1/4 lbs. zucchini
- 1 cup part-skim ricotta
- 1/4 cup parmesan
- 1 egg
- 1/4 cup fresh spinach, chopped
- 2 tablespoons fresh basil, chopped
- 1/4 teaspoon nutmeg
- 1/4 teaspoon salt
- 1/8 teaspoons black pepper
- 1 1/2 cups jarred marinara sauce
- 2/3 cup mozzarella, shredded
- 2 tablespoons parmesan, shredded
- 2 teaspoons olive oil
- 1/2 teaspoon black pepper
- Fresh basil, to garnish

Preparation:

1. At 375 degrees F, preheat your oven.
2. Cut the whole zucchini into thin strips using a potato peeler to get 60 slices.

3.   Mix black pepper, spinach, egg, salt, nutmeg, basil, spinach, parmesan and ricotta in a bowl.
4.   Spread marinara sauce in a 9x13 inches baking dish.
5.   Place two zucchini slices on a working surface in a cross.
6.   Add a tablespoon filling at the centre of this cross and wrap the zucchini slices around.
7.   Place the wraps in the casserole dish and drizzle olive oil, black pepper, salt and remaining cheese on top.
8.   Bake the ravioli for 30 minutes in the preheated oven.
9.   Serve warm.

Serving Suggestion: Serve the ravioli with pita bread and chili sauce.

Variation Tip: Add mashed sweet potatoes to the filling.

Nutritional Information Per Serving:

Calories 338 | Fat 24g |Sodium 620mg | Carbs 58.3g | Fiber 2.4g | Sugar 1.2g | Protein 5.4g

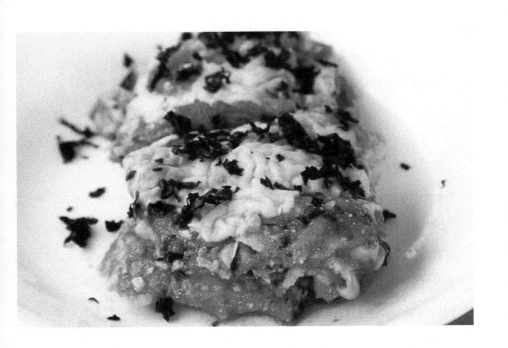

Cauliflower Salad

Prep Time: 5 minutes.

Cook Time: 0 minutes.

Serves: 4

Ingredients:

- 4 cups cauliflower florets
- 1 tablespoon Tuscan fantasy seasoning
- 1/4 cup apple cider vinegar

Preparation:

1. Toss cauliflower with seasoning and apple cider vinegar in a bowl.
2. Serve.

Serving Suggestion: Serve the cauliflower salad with lemon wedges.

Variation Tip: Add chopped mushrooms and bell pepper to the salad as well.

Nutritional Information Per Serving:

Calories 93 | Fat 3g |Sodium 510mg | Carbs 12g | Fiber 3g | Sugar 4g | Protein 4g

Tofu Spinach Sauté

Prep Time: 10 minutes.

Cook Time: 10 minutes.

Serves: 4

Ingredients:

- 1/4 cup onion, chopped
- 1/4 cup button mushrooms, chopped
- 8 ounces tofu, pressed and chopped
- 3 teaspoons nutritional yeast
- 1 teaspoon liquid aminos
- 4 cups baby spinach
- 4 grape tomatoes, chopped
- Cooking spray

Preparation:

1. Sauté mushrooms and onion with oil in a skillet for 3 minutes.
2. Stir in tofu and sauté for 3 minutes.
3. Add liquid aminos and yeast then mix well.
4. Stir in tomatoes and spinach then sauté for 4 minutes.
5. Serve warm.

Serving Suggestion: Serve the tofu with kale salad.

Variation Tip: Add boiled couscous to the mixture.

Nutritional Information Per Serving:

Calories 378 | Fat 3.8g |Sodium 620mg | Carbs 13.3g | Fiber 2.4g | Sugar 1.2g | Protein 5.4g

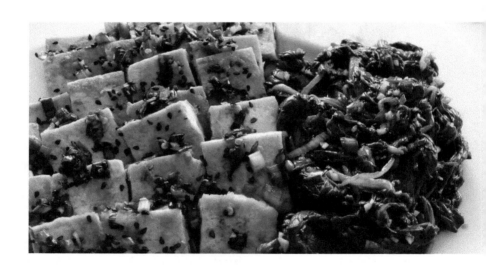

Zucchini Lasagna

Prep Time: 15 minutes.

Cook Time: 24 minutes.

Serves: 4

Ingredients:

- 6 ounces crumbled tofu
- 1 garlic clove, minced
- 1 tablespoon dried parsley flakes
- 1 tablespoon dried basil
- 1/8 teaspoons salt
- 1 can diced tomatoes, drained
- 3/4 cup 1% cottage cheese, shredded
- 3 ounces mozzarella cheese, shredded
- 1 tablespoon dried parsley flakes
- 2 tablespoons egg, beaten
- 2 small zucchini squash

Preparation:

1. At 350 degrees F, preheat your oven.

2. Cut the whole zucchini into thin slices using a potato peeler.

3. Sauté tofu with garlic, parsley, basil, and salt in a cooking pan until golden brown.

4. Stir in tomatoes, egg and parsley then cook for 4 minutes.

5. Spread a layer of thin zucchini slices at the bottom of a casserole dish.
6. Top these slices with half of the tofu mixture.
7. Mix cottage cheese with mozzarella cheese in bowl.
8. Drizzle 1/3 of the cheese mixture over the tofu filling.
9. Repeat the zucchini layer and top it with the remaining tofu mixture.
10. Add 1/3 of the cheese mixture and add another layer of zucchini on top.
11. Drizzle remaining cheese on top and bake for 20 minutes in the oven,
12. Serve warm.

Serving Suggestion: Serve the lasagna with the spinach salad.

Variation Tip: Add crispy fried onion on top for better taste.

Nutritional Information Per Serving:

Calories 304 | Fat 31g |Sodium 834mg | Carbs 21.4g | Fiber 0.2g | Sugar 0.3g | Protein 4.6g

Vegetable and Egg Casserole

Prep Time: 15 minutes.

Cook Time: 30 minutes.

Serves: 6

Ingredients:

- 6 eggs
- 1 cup egg whites
- 1 ¼ cup cheese, shredded
- 16 ounces bag frozen spinach
- 2 cups mushrooms, sliced
- 1 bell pepper, diced

Preparation:

1. At 350 degrees F, preheat your oven.
2. Beat egg with egg whites, cheese, spinach, mushrooms and bell pepper in a bowl.
3. Spread this egg mixture into a casserole dish.
4. Bake this casserole for 30 minutes in the oven.
5. Serve warm.

Serving Suggestion: Serve the casserole with cauliflower salad.

Variation Tip: Top the casserole with onion slices before cooking.

Nutritional Information Per Serving:

Calories 341 | Fat 24g |Sodium 547mg | Carbs 36.4g |
Fiber 1.2g | Sugar 1g | Protein 10.3g

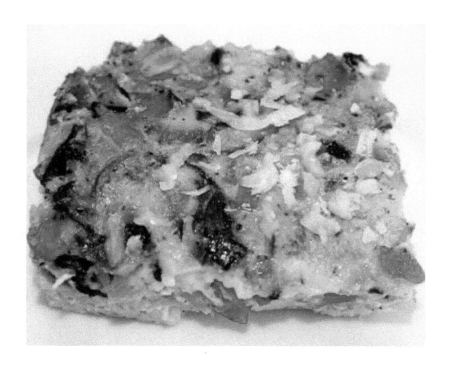

Lightning Source UK Ltd.
Milton Keynes UK
UKHW020645100621
385263UK00001B/166